Seven Movements to Keep you Healthy & Pain Free in the Office

Dan Tatton & John Sinclair

CONTENTS

ACKNOWLEDGMENTS

A special thank you goes out to Jennifer Tatton for providing her editing services for this book and Marie–Lise Norris for the cover design.

Also a special thank you to Carole Wood, our model, and to Juan Silva of JuanSilva Photography for the Movement section of the book.

WHY YOU NEED THIS BOOK

Our current approach to workplace wellness leaves a lot to be desired! As we know, we have more people working in offices and sitting behind a desk than any time in history. The technology that is meant to enhance our lifestyle has made life more efficient but much of it has come at a cost to the health of the human body. Some diseases and conditions attributed to our current office environments include lower back pain, neck pain, migraines and headaches, knee and hip pain, thoracic outlet syndrome, patella femoral syndrome, and carpal tunnel syndrome. Currently, we are failing to combat this very unnatural working environment effectively.

We are living in a crisis of inactivity made worse by our current work environments. The human body was not designed to sit for long periods of time. Nature calls for us to be standing, moving, and transitioning from position to position as we navigate the world around us. Moving is in fact, living. As we lose our ability to move we lose the ability to live and experience the world around us. Our current office environment can become part of the solution if we so choose.

Seven Movements aims to help you change the culture of your office environment from one of sedentary behaviors to one that is filled with meaningful movement. By providing you with simple targeted movements to help you combat the effects of too much sitting we will get you and your co-workers moving freely in your office again. We hope this is just the start to giving you the tools you need to create an office culture that promotes movement and creatively tackles the health issues that these office environments have caused. Let's get you thinking about exercise differently and start moving together!

1 THINK

The Problem

The office needs to become a place that nurtures movement, currently it is not. The problem with our current office environment is its sedentary design leads to pain. How effective are you when you are in pain? We spend much of our adult life working, many of us in offices. Our current office culture has us sitting and staring at screens for hours every day. This is not only completely unnatural but incredibly detrimental to our well-being.

We are then told that exercise is something you do after your work day when you go to the gym to "work out". Who really wants to "work" after a day at work? More on this later. The result has been an increase in pain and disease all the while creating a culture around movement that tells us that more pain is more gain and movement is for the gym not the office. Does anyone else see a problem with this? We do.

The human body was not designed to be seated for long periods of time. Movement is as natural to human beings as eating or breathing, both of which include movement we might add. It does seem counterintuitive that we have created work environments that require us to do the opposite of what our bodies were built to do. By building a work culture that does not value movement we have created a culture of inactivity that we try to solve by giving out gym memberships or handing out wellness pamphlets.

As personal trainers, we spend much of our time educating and coaching people how to move. The inability to move, specifically for office workers, generally presents itself as chronic pain and inflammation. Maybe you have experienced this in the form of lower back pain, headaches, neck pain, knee or hip pain, or countless other pains your body experiences due to lack of movement. This not only limits our effectiveness at work but outside of work as well. The most frustrating part is that most of these ailments are easily preventable.

Unfortunately, this problem then becomes cyclical because when you are in pain you hardly want to start moving more. While more movement is the cure, if you go to your doctor they will often provide you with a pill to numb the pain which does nothing to effect change to the root of the problem itself, lack of movement! This problem almost always manifests itself over time as pain. To better understand the problem we must look at what exactly pain is and where does it come from.

Why does it hurt?

So you are probably asking what all this pain talk has to do with movement at the office. To understand this we must first look at why we experience pain from not moving. Pain is an alarm system set up in the brain. In most cases it starts when there has been a traumatic or acute injury to the body. This could be physical or emotional. The brain will keep a memory of that pain , store it, and send a signal to warn the body that moving under those circumstances will not be a good thing.

Chronic pain is debilitating. It causes inflammation and we know that chronic inflammation is causing disease. One of the main reasons for experiencing chronic pain is the tissues of the body such as muscles, bones, fascia (the dense connective tissues that envelopes us) and nerves are not in synergy. That is, the body is not operating in harmony and is functioning in an unbalanced state. This causes the boney structures of the joints to misalign themselves relative to one another which overtime manifests itself as pain.

For example: the foot and ankle contain 33 joints, if a single joint is out of alignment the force that translates through the body while walking will not be properly dispersed throughout the body. That force can then cause pain in other areas of the body, most often the knee, hip, or back. Over time the body compensates for these imbalances and the dysfunction presents itself as chronic pain in multiple areas of the body. Think of the many times you hear your colleagues complain of a sore neck, headaches, a "bum" knee, an achy back, or tight shoulders? Many of these can be attributed to a lack of movement or rather holding positions like sitting for an extended period of time.

We need to remember what the human body is meant to do from a movement perspective. At a fundamental level it is meant to efficiently disperse ground reaction forces through the body imposed upon us from gravity and our own mass. That force passes through our connective tissue and if that system is out of balance that force will not pass through our body efficiently. This will result in a change in how the structures of the bones align with each other and over time result in even further dysfunction. What inherently will happen next is overuse in a dysfunctional position and an imbalance in the connective tissue and bony structures. The pain syndromes we listed earlier will ensue.

As the body compensates to get the job done (move) movement pathologies become more evident and the pain generally increases. We then spend time at doctors' offices for pills to numb the pain, massage therapists to relax tight muscles, or chiropractors to try to rebalance the joints. Unfortunately, these don't address the root of the problem, lack of purposeful movement.

What does this have to do with you sitting all day? Sitting puts our bodies' tissues out of balance. Remember our body's primary job is to mitigate the force of gravity. Let's take a quick look at how the act of sitting affects us negatively using our foot example from two paragraphs above.

Our glutes and hamstrings act like the bottom of our feet as we are sitting on them all day, our pelvis the foot and ankle while the lower back becomes the knee and so forth. As gravity acts on the body the tissues become unbalanced. The tensional balance between the connective tissues in the body are compromised and pain starts. That pain is not in the tissues but rather that alarm system set up in the brain to protect the tissues from further damage.

If you continue on this course the tissues will break down, joints will become misaligned and the body loses its ability to function. Compensation patterns arise in the form of "syndromes". Over time these compensation patterns cause us to lose the ability to move the joints that are supposed to move and stabilize the joints that are supposed to be stable. It has been proven that it takes as little as 15 minutes of sitting for the discs of the back to become dehydrated and the spine becomes compressed by gravity. Wow! Fifteen minutes.

Make no mistake all this sitting is killing us and if we don't start seeking movement as a solution *throughout* our workday we will not even start to begin solving this problem. We will spend countless hours in pain or at various doctors' offices. We need a new approach to getting people moving in the office.

Our current approach is failing

To their credit the business community has been trying to solve this problem. However, giving out gym memberships, building dark gyms in the basements of their buildings, and creating well designed pamphlets is not working. Many of these approaches treat movement as something you do outside of work rather than something you can do while you are working. I want you to take a moment to think how you spend your day. What are you doing when you send emails? Have meetings? Have lunch? We have developed a sitting culture around the workplace and if we want to truly change workplace wellness we need to address this.

Not only has the workplace failed, our entire attitude around exercise is failing. We tell people that it is no pain, no gain and they end up popping pills just to be able to keep moving without pain, after work of course. They then go down to the gym and "work out" sometimes dreading it more than they dread their work day. They are told of course they will benefit from all of this "sacrifice" by being blessed with health and strength. What they get is injuries, pain, and anxiety.

According to the CDC, anxiety, pain and injuries account for almost all work related illness and are a huge cost to businesses due to employees not being able to work. We need to start doing things differently and since the workplace is where we spend the majority of our day we need to start there. The workplace can be part of the solution.

The Solution

Fixing this problem is really not that complicated, however, it will take a change in mindset, a willingness to change the workplace culture, and an ability to look at the problem through a new lens. In other words, leadership! And it starts with you becoming a role model in your office by bringing movement into your own day as well as encouraging co-workers to create a culture of movement in your office. The good news is the human mind, body, and spirit crave movement just to survive and, when we keep it simple, we find the most consistent results. The workplace can be a catalyst to get people moving again and Seven Movements gives you a simple and effective way to get started.

We are going to show you how an investment of seven minutes can not only alter your perception of movement and exercise in the office but allow you to experience all the pain free movement in your day that you crave. We are going to show you how to connect to your exercise and give it purpose making it something you *want* to do rather than *have* to do.

Movement should be something we all want to do and we should be able to experience it doing the things we love. Whether it takes place in the gym, a pool, a track, a field, or anywhere else you like to enjoy movement is irrelevant. The point is that *you* enjoy it.

We want you to be a part of creating a culture of movement within your office by offering you a roadmap to help you get moving to prevent pain caused by sitting all day. Just by bringing more movement into your workspace you will prevent pain, increase your energy, and have more fun. Seven movements can change your life forever by celebrating movement and creating an environment that promotes movement within your workplace.

Just move

It all starts with movement. The movements in this book seek to get you up and moving IN the office effectively. They are also designed to specifically target and prevent the negative effects of sitting. Seven Movements and seven minutes will change your life forever. These movements are simple and effective and are the **first step** designed to allow you to experience movement in a positive way. Just because you have a desk job does not mean you are condemned to a lifetime of nagging pains and injuries. Take seven minutes and start benefitting from all the rewards of pain free movement right now.

Doing these movements consistently will mean a pain free and healthy work environment. They will also provide the capacity for maintaining strength and allow you to continue participating in the things you love after work. Perhaps that involves a gym, a team you compete with, or simply playing with your kids. Moving throughout our day is vitally important to our entire well-being as it gives us mental clarity, builds strength, burns calories, eliminates pain, and combats the harmful effects of sitting.

Moving does not need to be complicated nor painful so put down the magazines telling you how pain equals progress, turn off the television of screaming personal trainers belittling their clients, and just move baby! Experience new things and feel the joy of pain-free movement doing all of the things you love doing. Allow your workplace to be the catalyst of developing a new attitude towards movement and exercise. We are right here with you.

Changing the paradigm

To start experiencing movement in a positive way we need to start by changing the way we look at exercise and movement. The old paradigms of the past are no longer working and we need a new direction. We have to make movement an essential part of our day. Some of us spend the majority of our days inside the office so it is only natural to bring a culture of movement into that space.

The beautiful thing about it is that it is something our mind, body, and spirit craves. Modern day technology has given us the gift of not "having" to move for survival but allowing us to experience movement in ways that we enjoy. In other words instead of having to experience movements through strenuous tasks needed for survival as our ancestors did we can experience movement in a fun game of soccer or a hike in the mountains searching for the perfect view of a sunset.

The point is that we are moving and experiencing movement in a positive way. The seven movements in this book are the first step and are designed to give your body the capacity to enjoy movement in any form you like. They will empower you to experience pain free movement on your terms for the rest of your life. Help us bring this new paradigm to your place of work.

Our Current Paradigm

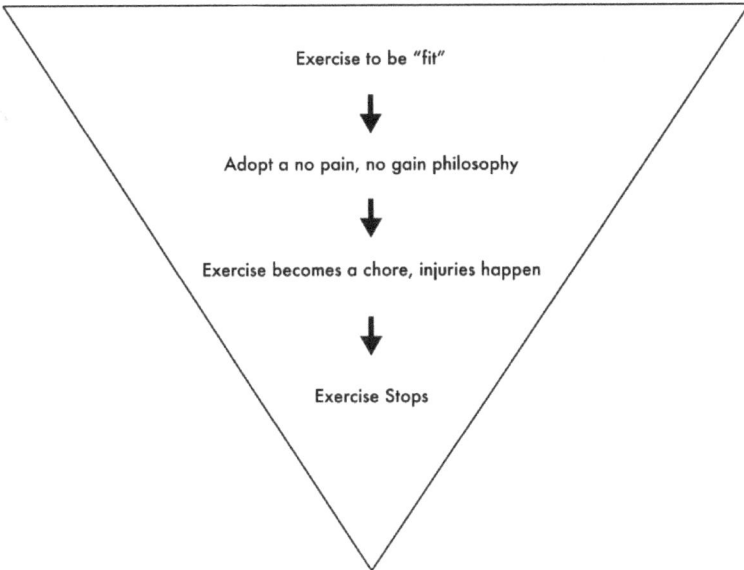

When we ask our average client about why he or she started an exercise program we generally get one of two answers: to lose weight or to "get fit". The second question we ask is what comes to mind when you hear the word "exercise"? And the same three words always come up: work, pain, and sweat. Now these are hardly words that would inspire a person to jump on the exercise program bandwagon.

As personal trainers, we have watched countless people with the goal of "getting fit" make it a chore to go to the gym because they feel exercise needs to be difficult to be effective. These people will spend countless hours in the gym staring at themselves in the thousands of mirrors to dwell on every tiny flaw in their body. Thousands of people join gyms in January and stick with their program until March before quitting from feeling more miserable, tired, and defeated than they started out. These people have bought into the message that in order to succeed they must "push through the pain" and that "pain equals progress". This type of message is not only unrealistic, but can lead to injury later on.

How did this happen? How did we turn something as beautiful

and necessary as movement into something we would rather not do? It started with advertising through the mainstream fitness industry that gave us such slogans as "no pain, no gain", that told people if they were not experiencing pain they were not working hard enough. To our dismay, this is still a strongly held belief amongst many who call themselves fitness professionals today. The way this image of exercise affects our psyche today is obvious.

We have TV shows with screaming "personal trainers" belittling those to work so hard they feel pain. People running on treadmills in so much pain they cannot even stand up straight, and worse yet, they are not even going anywhere! This type of exercise is not functional but fashionable.

This attitude is not only wrong but it will affect your ability to experience any movement in a positive way. So it is no surprise that when we say the word exercise most people immediately associate it with something they *have* to do rather than something they *want* to do. The end result is we are serving fewer people that truly need us. YOU!

There is nothing more tragic than watching someone have to stop doing something they love because it now causes them pain. It is even worse when that particular pain could be avoided by simply moving more at work. Most people don't realize they are not moving correctly until they start feeling pain and they are then told they need to be stronger. They go to the gym to strengthen weakness in the pursuit of pain relief. However, it doesn't work and generally lands them in the doctor's office where they are given a magic pill and told to get to the gym and start exercising. And the cycle continues.

We need to change this attitude as soon as we can. We know that these seven movements are the first step! We have been using these movements with all of our office clients and they move from improvements and changes in their posture to ultimately reversing their symptoms into pain free living and working. It is time that this becomes mandatory in our workplace and our lives.

The New Seven Movements Paradigm

Find some thing you love doing that involves movement "your why"

↓

Connect your Exercise to that thing you love doing

↓

Exercise to enjoy pain free movement for life

↓

Exercise Continues

In our new Seven Movements paradigm we look at exercise in a completely different way. We look at movement in the office as a vital part of keeping us in the condition to experience movement pain free while doing the activities we love. Our ancestors took care of their movement through everyday living. Our current work office environments have us moving as little as possible thus causing us a lot of pain and countless injuries. This is an incredibly unnatural environment for our bodies and we are seeing the affects.

Our view is we have been given the gift of being able to enjoy movement doing the things we love as we no longer have to move to hunt and forage or run from predators. Our exercise programs can be functional and efficient and this book gives you a program that will allow you to eliminate pain, reduce injury, feel stronger, and allow you to continue experiencing pain free movement for life.

Anyone can do these movements whether you are young or old. Give yourself seven minutes and we will give you a lifetime of pain free movement. The more frequently you invest those seven minutes, the healthier and happier your body will be.

When you give exercise purpose you will not only view exercise in a positive light but you will be astonished at the progress you make. You will begin to wonder how it is you are losing weight, having more energy, and getting stronger. Exercise will no longer be work, it will be the expression of movement it is meant to be. You will eliminate the harmful effects of sitting. Pain and weakness will never be the reason you don't participate in the things you love doing. You will be empowered with the ability to exercise on your terms.

Finding your *Why*: Reconnecting to Movement

Implementing Seven Movements in the office will allow you to connect with your *why*. When we start a new exercise program with someone we ask them to tell us their *why*. What is their purpose for wanting to exercise? Finding your *why* allows you to connect with your movement and it becomes much more than just exercise. It gives your exercise purpose beyond "getting fit" and allows you to connect with your true goals.

Finding your why is simple. Just ask yourself: What is it I love doing that involves movement? This will allow you to connect instantly to why it is you love moving in the first place. Do you enjoy playing with your kids or grandkids? Kayaking? Do you enjoy golfing without back pain? Is it the reward of a beautiful garden filled with fresh produce and lush flowers? Being fit is nothing more than an outcome of finding your *why* from applying the solutions in this book.

Seven Movements will keep you pain free in the office and enhance your ability to connect to even more movement outside the office setting. Exercise is about learning to move, connecting with your body, and giving you the ability to do the things you love without pain or injury. The movements you do in the office can combat those negative effects of sitting and keep you moving pain free for life.

As function relates to purpose, sometimes as in sitting, we endure positions that exceed the tolerance for the body's tissues. The burden on these tissues results in pain signals from the body and the brain. We will show you how to build resilient tissues that will allow you to stay healthy and pain free in the office. It is time to build strength, eliminate pain, and reduce your chance of injury.

Creating a culture of movement at work

The business community has, very recently, started to recognize not only the importance of wellness in the office but have been able to tie it to workplace performance. To be your best self you need to be healthy. Something as small as experiencing lower back pain throughout the day can affect your work performance negatively.

The problem is the way business has attacked this problem has been to simply hand out gym memberships or provide "resources" for their employees to pursue, generally outside of work hours. Unfortunately, workers have only become more sick, more tired, and more injured than ever before. This will manifest into anxiety about performance. Anxiety is the single greatest reason for missed work according to the Center for Disease Control.

The solutions companies have come up with seem reasonable: give out gym memberships, build a gym, design some pamphlets, make some external resources available, etc. While these things are not terrible, they hardly do anything to help create a culture of movement within the organization. First of all not everyone enjoys going to the gym, now some of our personal trainer friends might say "suck it up and it takes sacrifice to take care of your health". A false choice spouted by many gym managers today.

Our answer is simple: adopt the new Seven Movements Paradigm of looking at exercise by finding things you love doing that involve movement. Allow yourself to enjoy movement again by trying new things you enjoy doing. You will find that by preventing pain and injury at work you will be able participate and enjoy other activities that keep you moving outside of work.

Let us also take a look at where many organizations put their own gyms: usually in the basement or some less desirable location in your building and usually set up for a body builder working out in the 1980's. Not a really inviting place to go for most people if you ask us. Most North American facilities or gyms are set up to do things the vast majority of Americans refuse to go to. According to recent stats only 12% of Americans even have a gym membership. Something should be telling us that the environments are not meeting peoples "WHY".

This book aims to help you take the first step in creating a culture and environment of movement within your organization. Providing you with efficient and useful movements to keep you pain free at your desk is just the beginning. We hope it gets you talking about other ways you might incorporate movement in your day.

What if your gym became a meeting place? What if your gym didn't look like a body builder's hangout from the 1980's and became a wellness centre? What if walking meetings became the norm? What if your wellness centre became the hub of your organization? What if every hour you took a brain break and incorporated our program at your desk? Or played with a balloon with a coworker? How might that change the overall wellness of the people you work with? How about their performance and morale?

Seven Movements gives you the simple start you need to start developing a workplace culture that values movement and well-being. All of this is included in the **Take 7 Program**. By simply implementing Seven Movements you are becoming part of the solution to creating a culture of movement at your office.

Bringing movement to the workplace will change lives and inspire others to follow your lead. When moving at your desk becomes the norm instead of a rarity you are going to know you helped bring a culture to your organization that literally saves lives.

This book acts as step one in our **Take 7 Program**. Check out our website to see the next steps you can take in bringing a culture of movement to your office including getting **Take 7 Certified.**

The Take 7 Program looks at bringing creative solutions to your workplace that fit in your specific environment to get people moving and experiencing movement while doing the things they love at the place they work.

For information on bringing Dan and John into your organization, getting Take 7 Certified or to start a Take 7 program in your office you can contact us through our website.

2 EAT

This book is about movement but it would be hard to justify writing a book about movement if we didn't touch on the importance of diet on overall well-being. Eating well is the foundation of health and without a proper diet you certainly will not be moving well. For those who are not eating well or are confused about what they should eat, this will be the most important part of this book.

What should we eat to be healthy? It seems like such a simple question doesn't it? So why then does it provoke the most complicated answers? This book aims to keep things simple and practical. Eating well can be broken down into three foundation principles that, if followed, will lead to a healthy and balanced diet.

With office workers it often comes down to the much maligned lunch. What do I eat? What is easy? What if I eat out a lot. Many of the answers to these questions will become extremely evident once applying the principles below.

When it comes to your diet, if you don't apply these principles, it really doesn't matter what diet plan or nutritional "expert" you are following, you are unlikely to find success. Not only will you continue to manipulate your body chemistry making each future attempt to lose weight more and more difficult, but you are going to waste your time doing it. The following principles will form your base of healthy eating and, by mastering them, you will be in a position to understand your diet, food, your body, and what works best for you. Your body will then be in a position to adopt new healthy changes to your diet on your terms. This is the key ingredient in creating new habits.

Principle One: Just Eat Real Food

We were introduced to the term JERF by a man named Sean Croxton who runs the website *Underground Wellness*. JERF means to Just Eat Real Food. While this principle may seem like common sense, it has been all but abandoned by many experts who push miracle products, elimination of entire foods groups, mailing pre-packaged food to you (this is just weird), and completely neglecting the quality of the food they are telling people to eat. There is a big difference in the quality of foods we see in pre-packaged meals and fresh real food we prepare ourselves. We challenge you to look around at lunch time and see how much real food is being eaten. A big line up at the lunchroom microwave should give you a hint.

Before starting any healthy eating plan or "diet" you would be wise to make sure it takes into account the quality of the food you are putting into your body. In order to move, your body needs fuel and, without considering the quality of that fuel, you will be starting any diet from a faulty base. Might you lose weight from some wildly concocted diet or one that severely restricts your caloric intake? Sure. However, long term success isn't likely when we don't consider our body's needs or the quality of the food we choose to put into it.

Many of you may have experienced the yo-yo like effect of these diets that promise rapid and permanent weight loss. The diet industry is a multi-billion dollar industry and it is only going to make money if you are not successful. If their diets worked, you wouldn't need to spend money on them anymore. They operate on the same principle as gambling. The first time you try it, you lose some weight, and then they know you will continue to spend money on diets hoping you will "win" again.

Although we have had clients try to convince us that rice crackers and honey nut cheerios are real food, we all know intuitively what real food is. Real food nourishes us and gives us energy. Real food grows from healthy soil or feeds on healthy plants. Real food we can grow ourselves and it generally isn't found in the frozen food aisle.

The problem with real food is that corporations cannot patent it and sell to you like they can their "proprietary products" although some are trying. Any so called nutritional "expert" that is not talking about real food and the quality of foods you are putting in your body is wasting your time. *Just Eat Real Food* and you will begin to see how much energy your body will have for daily movement; it will change your life forever.

Action Steps

1. Get to know your farmer and where your food comes from. Ask them questions and learn about the steps your farmer is taking to ensure you get real food on your table. A great place to get to know your farmer is at your local farmers market. Start a real food challenge at your workplace and post recipes around the office

2. Start cooking. A sure fire way to know that your are just eating real food is by controlling the ingredients yourself.

3. Plan your meals. There is nothing worse than ending your workday and not knowing what it is you are going to eat. Of course your are going to go for fast food. Plan a weeks worth of meals in advance, do your shopping, and stick to it.

4. Check out Real Food Friday on our Blog at www.sevenmovements.com where we will be sharing real food recipes perfect for you and your family every Friday.

Principle Two: Recognize that your optimal dietary requirements are unique

This is yet another simple principle that so many miss or choose to ignore. Your optimal dietary requirements are unique. There is no perfect diet that will fit every person on earth, period. We are all uniquely different on the inside just as we are on the outside. Why is this ignored?

Promoters of diets won't tell people that their diet will only work with certain segments of the population; that would be cutting off a large portion of their possible market share. It is much easier to tell you they have a one sized fits all solution. This is simply not true.

Understanding this principle will allow you to make sound personal decisions about your diet for the rest of your life. Without this understanding we can easily be sold on cheap quick fixes, get pulled into diet groups, and never understand why we are the only one not losing weight. If we do not recognize our uniqueness we will spend our lives following other people's diets instead of working to find our own personal optimal diet.

Our differences extend beyond our physical appearances. When the next celebrity comes out with a book or magazine article promoting a diet because it made them feel great we should not expect that it should do the same for us. In fact, we should understand it probably won't. Understanding this enables us to make better decisions about our diet choices. Empower yourself through the simple recognition that you are unique and need to find your own way. And to find your own way we must move on to principle three.

Action Steps

1. Throw away your magazines. Seriously, get rid of them. This way you won't be tempted when the next celebrity comes out with their own miracle diet. Nor will you be distracted by the next "study" that tells you that eating eggs are good for you followed by next weeks edition with a "study" that tells you eating eggs is bad

for you. We have a list of recommended reading on our website if you wish to dive deeper into the subtleties of your diet.

2. Write these words down, " I am unique". Post them everywhere. Remind yourself constantly that you are a unique individual that will empower yourself through your own knowledge. Only you know what makes you feel best and don't forget it.

Principle Three: Learn to listen to your body

This principle is something that is going to help you drown out much of the noise coming from celebrities, nutritional "experts", and diet books. We often get it from all angles. Eat vegan! Eat Paleo! Follow Atkins! Follow South Beach! The list is endless. Experts, friends, and even family will often tell you that their way of eating is the only way that is good for you. By taking time to learn to listen to your body you will be able to know definitively whether or not what you are eating is working for you. You will know because you will connect how you feel to what you are eating.

As trainers we have seen people on all types of diets from vegans to people following Atkins that made them feel tired and awful. On the flip side, we have had clients who moved to those same diets and it changed their lives for the better. This simply highlights how vital it is to learn to listen to your body as it will respond uniquely to how you eat and how you move. Not only that but your bodies requirements may change over time depending on what kind of lifestyle you are leading.

So many people are not only disconnected from the food they eat but from their own bodies as well. Lack of energy, indigestion, irritability, stress, soreness and so many more ailments are accepted as a normal part of life. It does not have to be this way, it is time to empower ourselves by learning to listen to our bodies. Our bodies have so much to tell us.

Your body will tell you which foods are giving you lasting energy and which are giving you a quick boost followed by a crash. It will tell you which foods make you feel tired and irritable and which foods give you a sense of strength and clarity. Many people will notice the obvious intolerances to food but many miss the subtleties. It is time to start really listening, if you are eating like your nutritional "expert" says you should and feel horrible, you need to listen to your body and try something else. Sometimes trial and error is the only way but remember you must also take into account principles one and two. Trust us, it will be worth it.

As you learn to listen to your body you will start to tune out all of the arguing going on between the diet experts and daily conflicting research because you will know what makes you feel at your best and what doesn't. When that friend drops by to tell you about his/her latest diet, you can smile and nod while knowing you are going to stick with what works for you. Embracing this principle will empower you to make decisions based on how food makes *you feel* rather than how someone else tells you it should make you feel.

Action Steps

1. Test test test. Recognize how you feel after you eat. Do you feel full? Do you feel hungry? Do you feel like napping? Full of energy? All of these symptoms could be a result of what you are eating.

2. If you have foods you suspect are bothering your digestion or making you feel poorly start by eliminating them for two weeks at a time. Do you feel a difference?

3. Bring some variety into your diet. Stagger the types of foods you are eating and you will be able to recognize the subtleties of how certain types of foods are making you feel.

Allow these principles to be your measuring stick before attempting any diet plan. Remember that there are many excellent nutritional experts out there that are ready to guide you through this process should you require it. But be sure their practices are rooted in these principles as they are unchanging. We hope you can take them and free yourself to make the choices you need to make to feel better and live healthier. Good luck and happy eating!

3 MOVE

Movement is life. In this section of the book we are going to give you seven simple movements that will help you combat sedentary behavior in the office, primarily sitting. They are going to help you avoid injury, keep your joints healthy, and change the way you view the word "exercise" forever. When speaking with people who work in the office setting, we often hear complaints of aching joints and sore backs. As personal trainers there is nothing that challenges us more than seeing someone in pain due to an inability to move freely. Know that it does not have to be this way.

Movement need not be complicated to be effective. The exercise industry has done a terrible job of promoting this concept. Our bodies have been designed to move from the beginning of time. In the diet section of this book, we talked about recognizing our individuality and now we need to realize that our movements might also need to be unique. We are going to look at the very fundamentals of what keeps our bodies moving successfully (meaning without pain). We want to give you simple tools that you can use throughout your day in the office setting. Yes, it is time to start moving *in* the office.

We have talked about how sedentary behaviors are the root cause of most pain being felt in offices around the world. We have also talked about how simply promoting activity "outside" of work is not addressing this issue, in fact, the pain the office is causing us is affecting our ability to move outside of work as well. We are going to give you the first steps you need to get moving at the office as well as the ability to start a culture of movement within your office setting. Are you ready to begin?

These seven simple movements will help you gain the freedom from pain that comes from extensive sitting, the potential to burn calories, and make you a more effective worker. When you experience freedom from pain this will allow you to pursue movement(exercise) in other facets of your life. This can mean joining a gym, joining a new club, or simply playing with your children daily. Let your passions to guide you to a stronger and healthier body that will keep you moving for life.

Allow us to guide you through these movements, perform them once every hour at your desk. It is time to TAKE 7 and start moving again!

1. Back Triangle Stretch

Being seated in front of the computer will deform the tissues into a forward head posture that causes headaches and neck pain. This seated position will also elevate and tilt the shoulder blades causing migraines, thoracic outlet syndrome and carpal tunnel syndrome.

We perform this movement to create length in the neck as well as to pull the shoulders down and back and to lengthen the tissues in the chest reducing these negative consequences of sitting.

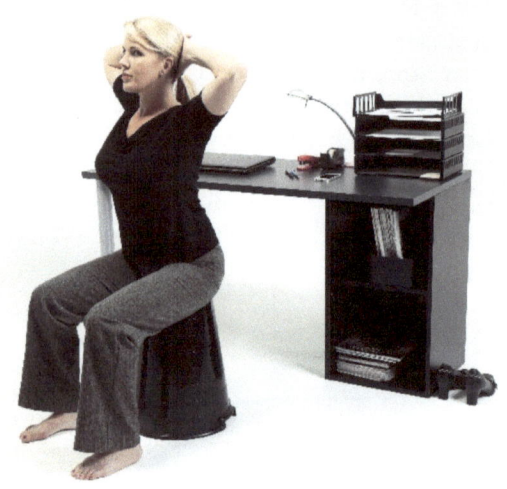

Coaching tips

"Interlock fingers behind head"
"Stretch elbows apart to form triangle"
"Head reaches up to the sky"

2. Seated Sky Reach

Sitting can cause compression of the thoracic(upper) spine causing a forward head posture which deforms the tissues in the upper back making them plastic and less elastic. Typing shortens the tissues in the arms further compressing joints.

This movement builds length in the upper back (thoracic spine) as well as lengthens the tissues in the arms and neck thus lessening the compression on these joints.

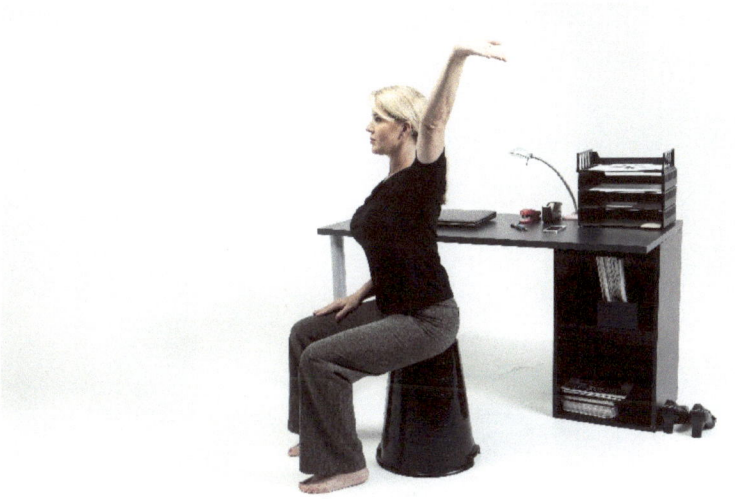

Coaching Tips

"Single arm Palm Stretch to the Sky"
"Hand Position: is like holding a tray with a bowl of Soup"

3.   Single Leg Hammy Rock

When sitting you smash the sliding surfaces of the connective tissue together causing them to glue together. This results in low back pain. It is crucial that we unglue the hamstrings and pump water into the tissues.

This movement will create elasticity, pump water into the connective tissue, and create length in the posterior part of the lower body preventing lower back pain.

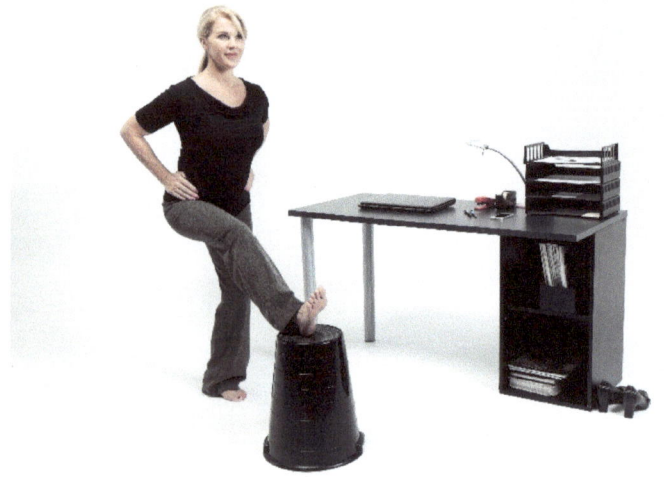

Coaching Tips

"Elevate Leg"
"Pull toes to nose and push heel away from body"
"Hinge hips"
"Stand tall"
"Lower hips towards carpet"
"Rock the Trunk slowly"

4. Wide Stance Booty Shift

Being in a seated position we immobilize the pelvis by squashing many of the tissues surrounding it causing them to become glued which quickly manifests as lower back pain.

This movement will unglue the hamstrings from the inner thigh tissues known as the adductors. This will also help "De-couple" the hips to create more space and movement in the Sacroiliac (SI) joint which will greatly reduce back pain.

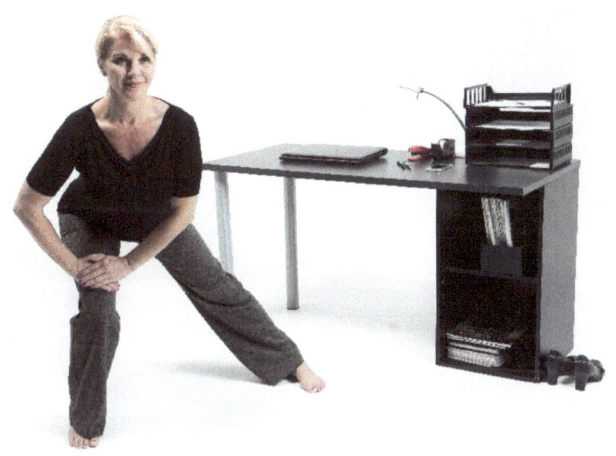

Coaching Tips

"Hinge hips and shift weight to one side"
"Full foot contact on floor"
"Feel a stretch in the inner thigh"
"Be sure to do both sides"

5.   Standing Bow Position

The sitting position causes compression in the lower back by taking our spine into too much flexion.

This slow and subtle movement will help decompress the spine by creating extension in the lumbar spine. This will help bring extension back into the pelvis, hip, and lower back and unload the locked muscles of the back reducing pain.

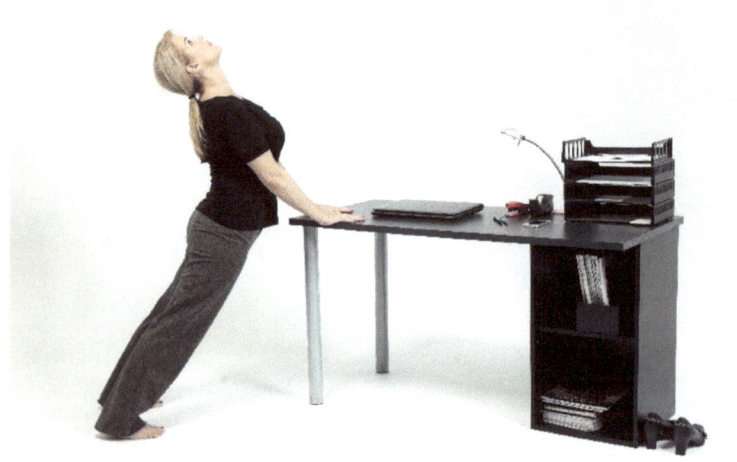

Coaching Tips

"Hands on desk"
"Feet flat"
"Push hips forward"
"Pull shoulders back"
"Look up to the sky"

6. Twisting C Leg Swings

Being seated eliminates rotation from our joints reducing our ability for optimal motion when we do get up and move. These compressed joints become less mobile and pain quickly shows up. In order to create space in joints (decompress) we need to introduce rotation into our everyday activity.

This movement introduces rotation to your daily routine optimizing the mobility of your joints. Rotation is the most efficient movement in the body and is largely forgotten in typical exercise programs. Plus its fun!

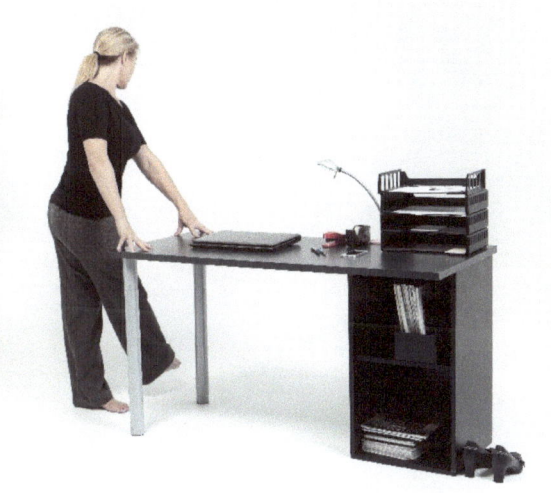

Coaching Tips

"Hands on table"
Swing leg inwards and then outwards"
"Single Right Leg balance-Draw a C with the toes back and forth"
"Single Left Leg Balance-Draw a reverse C with toes back and forth"
"This is a controlled movement"

7.   Half Stance Arm Stretcher

Sitting chronically shortens and dehydrates the tissues of the body.

This movement will enhance all of your joints and rehydrate the tissues by creating rotation in the body while simultaneously lengthening the arms, abdomen, hips and lower leg.

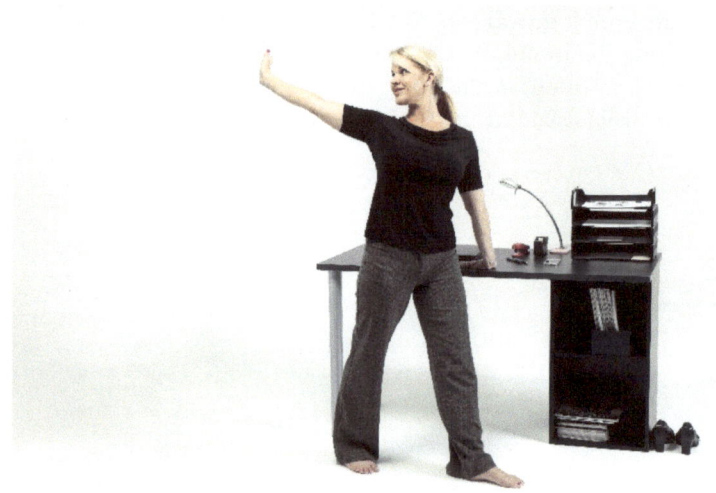

Coaching Tips

"Palm flat on desk"
"Inside leg staggered forward"
"Reach back with fingers pointed to sky"
"Palm reaches away from body"
"Be sure to do both sides"

Thank you so much for being a part of Seven Movements.

This is just the start of your seven movement journey. To take the next steps and join us to become TAKE 7 certified contact us at

www.sevenmovements.com

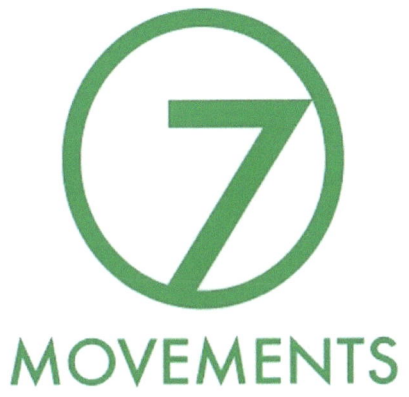

ABOUT THE AUTHORS

John Sinclair

When Dan Tatton asked me to collaborate on this project I could not have been more excited. We both realized that the fitness industry was moving in the opposite direction of where we are needed most. While other personal trainers search for the newest and craziest exercises, Dan and I noticed that we need to share the simplest and most effective movements to help people enjoy the activities that they are currently doing. It was becoming ridiculous to me that my clients were joining a gym just to regain strength and stamina to be able to do the things they loved to do outside of the gym.

In an effort to help people deal with their complaints we created this book to provide solutions to your problems. These problems may include back and joint pain, chronic headaches, fibromyalgia and other musculoskeletal disorders. We want you to have the ability to do what you love, when you want to do it and for as long as possible. These movements that we have created for you are simple, replicable and most importantly they work!

I would be remiss if I didn't thank my mentors, friends and clients and of course family. The people that helped me become the coach I am today. My friend and former colleagues Jeff Thirsk and Ricky Tran, you have always supported me in any endeavor I have taken on. All the coaches and trainers I have worked alongside. Because of you I am who I am. To my clients, Thank you. For your trust and your friendship. The relationships we have cultivated have provided the most everlasting memories and experiences. I will always cherish the time we spend together. Michol Dalcourt, Scott Hopson, Rodney Corn, Bobby Cappuccio, Richard Boyd, and the entire faculty of PTA Global and Institute of Motion. Your mentorship is crucial to my development and continual search to be a better coach and educator. A special thanks to Ian ODwyer who has helped me simplify movement and has inspired me to include his concept of Mobilizers into this book.

To my family. Lisa, my wife, my partner in life. Without your continual support I would not be here today writing a book about experiences and solving peoples problems. We have endured, evolved, and experienced so much together. I thank you for your selflessness and helping me achieve my dreams. My mother Kate, brothers Jeremy and Jesse and sister Caitlin. Thanks for your love. I cherish every moment we get to spend with one another. I miss you.

And to you the reader. Thanks for taking the first step to experiencing life changing movement with the solutions we have included in this book.

Good luck. I know that you will be able to experience the world the way we are designed to so that you may move, play and be healthy and happy.

This truly is the first step to a revolution of movement. Are you ready to take the first step?

Dan Tatton

Partnering with John Sinclair on this book has been an incredible experience. As personal trainers we want the world to experience more movement. Technology has given us the gift of choosing how we want to experience movement on a daily basis. Let's take advantage of that and do what we love to do.

This book is an effort to give you the simplest most effective tools you need to combat the sedentary nature of the current office environment. It aims to flip the " no pain, no gain" attitude on its head and allow you to build strength, eliminate pain, and begin moving with ease.

The reason I started writing this book was to help those that want to find health. It is the first step of our Take 7 Program that aims to give you the simplest tools you need to experience movement in a positive way. By making movement WITHIN the office environment so simple and so accessible you are part of a growing movement of people who are starting to change the way we look at workplace wellness.

Thank you for being a part of an exercise revolution that brings a culture of movement into your office and changes the way people think about exercise at work. You are the leaders that will bring health back to one of the places we spend most of our time and in doing so you will be the leaders that turned the workplace into a place that enhanced our health, rather than took away from it.

Four years ago I set out to create an exercise program that was connected to your passion, easy and convenient to do, and supplemented the movement you already love to do. John was the perfect partner as he is the most brilliant movement specialist I have had the honor of seeing in action. Together, I knew we could change the way people look at exercise forever.

Writing this book has been a dream come true for me and I would like to thank all those that helped make it a reality. There are too many to list but you know who you are and all of you inspire me everyday.